Distribution, publication, and copying in any form are prohibited and subject to damages.

TEN HYPNOSES

Copying, publishing, and sharing with third parties are only permitted with the written consent of the author. Please observe the notes on copyright and usage.

Distribution, publication, and copying in any form are prohibited and subject to damages.

Copying, publishing, and sharing with third parties are only permitted with the written consent of the author. Please observe the notes on copyright and usage.

Distribution, publication, and copying in any form are prohibited and subject to damages.

Ingo Michael Simon

TEN HYPNOSES

10
Grief Work

Copying, publishing, and sharing with third parties are only permitted with the written consent of the author. Please observe the notes on copyright and usage.

Distribution, publication, and copying in any form are prohibited and subject to damages.

© 2024 Ingo Michael Simon
All rights reserved.
Independently published
www.ingosimon.com

Important Notes for Urgent Attention:
The contents of this book are based on the practical experiences of the author with hypnosis applications and psychotherapy in a trance state. Although the author has strived for the utmost care, errors or misunderstandings in the presentation cannot be completely excluded. Therapeutic work with people and the application of hypnosis are solely the responsibility of the hypnotist. It cannot be ruled out that parts of this book may be misunderstood or that the application of a presented procedure may cause an undesirable reaction in the client. The author also assumes no co-responsibility if work with a client is carried out with reference to the statements in this book.

The Author:
Ingo Michael Simon studied psychology and education and is a hypnotherapist with practices in southwestern Germany and Switzerland. With the help of hypnosis-supported psychotherapy, he primarily treats people with persistent psychological conditions. His practice focuses on anxiety disorders, pathological compulsions, and psychosomatic illnesses. His therapeutic offerings mainly include classical and modern hypnosis applications and the dreamland therapy he developed himself.

Copying, publishing, and sharing with third parties are only permitted with the written consent of the author. Please observe the notes on copyright and usage.

Distribution, publication, and copying in any form are prohibited and subject to damages.

Notes on Copyright and Usage

Copying, publishing, and sharing with third parties is prohibited and only permitted with the written consent of the author. Please observe the following copyright and usage guidelines.

This work has been carefully crafted and created to the best of the author's knowledge and personal experience. It comprises text templates and application guidelines for professional hypnosis sessions. The author is a licensed psychotherapist with extensive experience in psychotherapy, coaching, and personal training using hypnotic techniques and methods. Nevertheless, the author and the publisher assume no liability for the accuracy of information, instructions, and advice, nor for any typographical errors. The author and publisher accept no responsibility or liability for the application of these texts and recommendations with clients or patients, nor for any potential consequences or unexpected reactions. It is expressly noted that the application of therapeutic and advisory techniques and formulations lies solely and entirely within the responsibility of the practitioner. This also applies to adherence to the boundaries of legally regulated medical and therapeutic practices. The fact that a book containing action proposals is freely available for sale does not imply that its application with clients or patients is permitted for everyone.

Distribution, publication, and copying in any form are prohibited and subject to damages.

Copying, publishing, and sharing with third parties are only permitted with the written consent of the author. Please observe the notes on copyright and usage.

Distribution, publication, and copying in any form are prohibited and subject to damages.

Table of contents

Introduction 9
#1 11
#2 16
#3 21
#4 27
#5 32
#6 37
#7 42
#8 47
#9 52
#10 57
Overview of All Titles in the Series "Ten Hypnoses" 62

Copying, publishing, and sharing with third parties are only permitted with the written consent of the author. Please observe the notes on copyright and usage.

Distribution, publication, and copying in any form are prohibited and subject to damages.

Copying, publishing, and sharing with third parties are only permitted with the written consent of the author. Please observe the notes on copyright and usage.

Introduction

The series "Ten Hypnoses" is very well known in Germany, Austria, and Switzerland as a collection of texts for therapeutic work and is used by numerous psychotherapeutic practices, doctors, therapists, coaches, and other helping professionals. I am pleased to now be able to offer these texts in other countries as well.

Most therapists have their own methods for inducing and deepening trance as well as for exiting trance. Therefore, I have focused on the main part of the hypnosis. The texts in this book can be integrated as the main part into any hypnosis process.

The texts in this collection use various hypnosis techniques. I will not explain these in detail, as I assume that users have the appropriate training. It is also not necessary to understand the exact structure or functioning of the different parts. The texts can simply be read aloud, and they will have their effect.

Decide for yourself which text best suits your client or patient at any given time. You can also combine passages from different texts. It is not about using all ten hypnoses in sequence. It is a selection of possibilities.

I want to emphasize that books cannot replace therapy. Psychotherapy or other therapeutic treatments involve much more. A careful diagnosis is the necessary basis for deciding on the use of methods, including whether hypnosis or one of my texts should be used. Even in this case, preparatory discussions, follow-up discussions during the session, and of course, a therapeutic concept for the sequence of sessions and the content approaches are essential parts of therapy. This cannot and should not be achieved with a collection of texts.

In any case, I wish you much success in your work and I am pleased if my text templates can contribute in a small way.

Ingo Michael Simon

#1

You have realized that it is now important to view your grief as a challenge ... ... that it is essential to embrace life again and continue to engage actively ... ... You have taken this remarkable step and said: Yes, I can do this ... ... I will get through this ... ... I will tackle life ... ... Many times, you have overcome difficult times ... ... with patience and perseverance, you have weathered challenging phases and then looked forward again, saying ... ... Yes, I can do this ... ... I will get through this ... ... I will tackle life ... ... It's truly amazing how well you can adopt this constructive attitude once more ... ...

... ... Many times, you have managed to see challenges as opportunities and tackled them courageously ... ... You know how to solve problems and take a big step forward ... ... You also know what it feels like to overcome challenges ... ... So, right now, you commit to doing it again ... ... You view grieving and the feeling of loneliness as challenges that you will soon overcome ... ...

First, think about what it means to be alone or to feel lonely ... ... You know both feelings, but from now on, it will be different ... ... Alone but not lonely ... ... Alone but not lonely ... ... You know inner silence and can experience it now if you focus on it ... ... This silence becomes greater and deeper the more you think about how often you feel lonely ... ... Right now, you think intensely about loneliness to experience the silence deeply ... ... It becomes quieter around you ... ... quieter within you ... ... With each breath, it becomes quieter around you ... ... quieter within you ... ... Every sound you hear seems far away and fades ... ...

... ... The silence spreads ... ... In this silence, you listen deeply within yourself ... ... Now ... ... You listen deeply within yourself ... ... Now ... ... And from this inner silence, a new thought arises ... ... a thought that helps you make new plans ... ... find new contacts and feel good ... ... If you listen carefully, you can hear your own thoughts quietly ... ... They speak to you ... ... They tell you about yourself ... ... You realize that in this silence, you can find a great opportunity ... ... the opportunity to take care of yourself, to feel your emotions more clearly and to have space ... ... Even in being alone, new space emerges for you and your needs ... ... for thoughts you often couldn't hear ... ... So listen and enjoy the space you can now fill ... ... Amazing how much space there is for yourself ... ... Space that you can finally use to find out what you want most ... ... which paths you can best take now ... ... You now see seclusion as a challenge to fill the space of silence ... ... You feel the urge to actively and creatively fill this free space ... ...

You rest within yourself, and thoughts arise that show you what you really need ... ... maybe contact with friends ... ... perhaps connection with family or relatives ... ... maybe something entirely different ... ... You recognize that what you experienced as loneliness was mainly unfulfilled space within you ... ... Space that feels unfulfilled because a person who was important to you has passed away ... ... It is the inner space that you can fill not only with memories but also actively ... ... with things that are important to you ... ... your free space ... ... You imagine the two words in large, bold letters: Loneliness and Free Space ... ... You realize that both words describe the same thing ... ... the space you can fill ... ... the space you want to fill ... ... the space you will fill ... ... And you start right away ... ...

Your thoughts are set on filling this free space with creative ideas and plans ... ... Your feelings are set on giving you confidence and hope ... ... Confidence and hope ... ... Your body is set on taking an active and strong posture immediately ... ... Your body knows that it must take on the activity ... ... because you can best fill your free space through actions ... ... The more active you are, the more you can see your free space as an opportunity ... ...

So, in your thoughts, you let the word loneliness become smaller ... ... The word loneliness becomes smaller and, at the same time, the word free space becomes larger ... ... The smaller the word loneliness becomes, the larger and bolder the word free space becomes ... ... Your body increasingly adopts this active posture, creating a feeling in you that you need to move ... ... Your thoughts become active and quicker ... ... Ideas and plans emerge ... ... Ideas and plans that enable you to quickly establish social contacts and interact with other people ... ... to enjoy the day together with them ... ... You experience the inner free space as a challenge, as a great opportunity ... ... You have a strong desire for activity ... ... a strong desire for renewal ... ... a strong desire for change ... ... You feel the activity in every cell of your body ... ... Instead of grief, you now place beautiful memories ... ... Instead of loneliness, you now place the desire for life ... ... beautiful memories and the desire for life ... ...

You can always take time to find your inner free space ... ... in peace and relaxation, with pleasant music, you can find the silence within you and thus repeatedly discover the free space within you that shows you how much room there is for a fulfilling life ... ... You make yourself comfortable whenever you want, and you immediately find the silence within you that gives you strength and confidence ... ...

#2

You have lost someone and have grieved a lot ... ... Grieving is important because it is the expression of a very significant feeling that accompanies every farewell ... ... But now it is time to let go of the sadness ... ... Today you decide to let go of the grieving and allow joy to come back into your life ... ... You have firmly resolved to do this, and we will walk this path together ... ... Letting go of grief and allowing joy to enter your life ... ... First, you make the inner decision to let go of your grief now ... ... You align all your thoughts with it ... ... Your thoughts are now focused only on this one goal ... ... to let go of your grief today ... ... Truly remarkable how quickly you can fully commit to this ... ... how well you succeed in already deciding to let go of your grief ... ... You are now letting go of as much of your grief as possible ... ... you are already letting go of a large part ... ... like setting down an old object that you no longer need ... ... You succeed now ... ... You let go of another piece of your grief ... ... just like that ... ... You are doing it right ... ... It truly works ... ...

...... Then your mind deals with letting go of the grief ...... Your mind knows that it is important to keep overcoming difficult times ...... to leave them behind ...... Your mind knows that you have grieved enough ...... Any further grieving would be clinging to a time that is too old ...... to a past that is no longer relevant ...... Your mind knows this and acts accordingly ...... Your mind aligns itself with letting go of your grief now ...... And to keep letting go of grief whenever it arises again ...... Your mind is sharp and clear ...... It decides with you and for you that you will let go of your grief now ......

...... Next, your deep emotions adjust to letting go of grief ...... your inner feelings that needed this grief until recently ...... until recently, but today your feelings adjust to letting go ...... Letting go of the grief ...... You succeed today even better than expected ...... Remarkable how directly and strongly you can actually set your mind to letting go of the grief ...... It truly works ...... It truly works today ......

...... Breathe deeply, because this aligns your body even more with letting go ...... Each exhale is like a liberation ... ... like letting go again ...... Breathe in ... and out ...... [In the client's breathing rhythm, extending the exhale slightly longer than the client's actual breath to slow their breathing. This enhances the suggestive effect.] ... Breathe in ... ... and slowly and long out ... ... in ... ... and slowly and long out ... ... in ... ... and out ... ... in ... ... and out ... ... in ... ... and out ... ... good ... ... You truly let go ... ... You are doing it right ... ... good ... ... Your body has understood this principle ... ... It has established it itself ... ... Your body lets go of your grief ... ... Perhaps you have already thought about the fact that emotions are stored much longer in the body than in the mind ... ... Your mind has already decided to let go ... ... That is good and important ... ... Your body has also decided to let go ... ... That is even more important ... ... Today it is crucial that your body has let go of the grief ... ...

... ... Now there is space for new things ... ... Free space for you ... ... Free space for joy and confidence in your life ... ... This is now possible again ... ... Joy can now return to your life ... ... Your mind allows you to feel joy again and let joy come back into your life ... ... So, you become open to new paths and new impulses ... ... open to new experiences ... ... Joy can enter your life again ... ... Now ... ... Joy can enter your life again ... ... Now ... ... Now ... ...

... Even your deep inner self ... ... your subconscious adjusts to joy ... ... to openness ... ... to new things ... ... to confidence ... ... to hope ... ... to discovering and allowing joy in your life again ... ... Truly remarkable how well you succeed in experiencing joy again now ... ... allowing and actually feeling joy ... ...

You succeed today even better than expected ... ... Remarkable how directly and strongly you can actually set your mind to letting go of the grief ... ... It truly works ... ... It truly works today ... ...

... ... Breathe deeply, because this aligns your body even more with allowing joy ... ... Each inhale is like a liberation ... ... like allowing joy again ... ... Breathe deeply in ... and slowly out ... ...

... ... [Here follows a sequence in the client's breathing rhythm, applying some "pressure" in the voice during the inhale to enhance the deep breathing. This enhances the suggestive effect.] ... ...

... ... Breathe deeply in ... ... and slowly out ... ... deeply in ... ... and out ... ... deeply in ... ... and out ... ... deeply in ...

… and out … … deeply in … … and out … … good … … You truly allow joy … … You are doing it right … … good … …

You realize once again that every inner truth can also become an outer truth … … Everything you can think and imagine can become reality immediately if you want it to be … … So, you want it with all your strength … … Letting go of grief and allowing joy … … Your body internalizes this and breathes actively for you tonight while you sleep … … With every inhale in your sleep tonight, you allow joy … … with every exhale, you let go of grief … … With every inhale in your sleep tonight, you allow joy … … with every exhale, you let go of grief … … just like now … …

#3

The following hypnosis session works with a combination of affirmation hypnosis and anchor technique. An affirmation is a short belief statement offered as a suggestion and can be used by the client as self-suggestion. An anchor is a trigger that evokes a specific feeling or thought. We work with the affirmation and simultaneously with an anchor in the form of a handy card with the printed phrase "I embrace life". This short phrase is an excerpt from the affirmation. We aim to help the client quickly adjust to letting go of grief and actively embracing life with the help of a "reminder card" when they notice that grief is holding them back in everyday life. We discuss this with the client before the session and prepare the reminder card. It can be a labeled business card or something similar. The card is prepared and given to the client. They can hold it loosely in their hand or place it on their body, for example on the solar plexus, during the hypnosis. The card should be carried by the client after the hypnosis, in their pants or jacket pocket. The main hypnosis part is deliberately kept very short to make the *affirmation very clear and establish it as a fundamental statement, as a new belief. The advantage of hypnosis is that the affirmation is more easily accepted by the client than in a conscious state. However, this hypnosis should not serve as the first session but should be introduced when the client has already gone through a certain processing stage.*

Imagine you are sitting in a cinema ... ... An old cinema, just like they used to be ... ... With thick, soft seats, covered in velvet ... ... Very soft seats ... ... Make yourself comfortable in a soft velvet seat ... ... You are all alone in this cinema ... ... The whole hall is empty and it is quiet, very, very quiet ... ... Look around a little in your cinema hall ... ... The floor is soft ... ... A very soft carpet ... ... Maybe a dark red ... ... a beautiful dark red ... ... The walls are covered with colored fabric ... ... Red and green ... ... red and green ... ... And from the ceiling hangs a huge chandelier, with many light bulbs and countless crystals ... ... It illuminates just enough for you to see everything clearly ... ... Make yourself very comfortable in your seat, make yourself feel good in your soft seat ... ... On the walls of the cinema hang small lanterns ... ... two or three on each side, left and right ... ... Small purple gas flames burn in them ... ... The screen far ahead is covered by a thick, heavy curtain ... ... A dark, heavy curtain covers the screen in this beautiful cinema ... ... It gradually gets darker and darker ... ... The light is dimmed and it gets darker and darker ... ... And you can become more comfortable and more relaxed within yourself ... ... The curtain slowly opens, the long, heavy, dark curtain gradually moves aside ... ... The curtain opens more and more to reveal your screen ... ... And it gets darker and darker, quieter and quieter ... ... The curtain opens more and more ... ...

The soft hum of the projector can be heard, the intro begins ... ... On the screen in front is a number ... ... a ten ... ... And as the intro runs, numbers count down from ten to zero ... ... I count with you and you can sink deeper with each number I mention ... ... ten ... ... nine ... ... eight ... ... seven ... ... six ... ... five ... ... four ... ... three ... ... two ... ... one ... ... the film is about to begin ... ... it's about to start ... ... it can begin now ... ... zero ... ... now it starts ... ... now it begins ... ... And on the screen in large, bold letters it says ... ...

I embrace life.

I understand death and farewell as part of my life

and am ready to let go of all the painful now.

I am ready to shape my life anew.

I embrace life.

You let the words resonate deeply within you and continue to look at the screen ... ... These words are there just for you ... ... It is your message ... ... You read them again ... ...

I embrace life.

I understand death and farewell as part of my life

and am ready to let go of all the painful now.

I am ready to shape my life anew.

I embrace life.

You know the crucial phrase ... ... I embrace life ... ... It is like a message to yourself ... ... I embrace life ... ... It is like a reminder ... ... I embrace life ... ... like a prompt that only you can give yourself ... ... I embrace life ... ...

You have this card with exactly this inscription, the card that holds your task ... ... I embrace life ... ... The card you feel between your fingers reminds you of it ... ... every day ... ...

... ... [Now ask the client to open their eyes and read the sentence while in trance. This reinforces the effect. Opening the eyes is a fractionation, but it can be done without specific announcement or counting. Everyone can open their eyes in trance. In a stable and deep trance, it is a bit cumbersome because the client is tired and sluggish. Just stay with suggestive encouragement until the eyes are opened and the card is read. If you prefer to initiate the fractionation by counting, you can certainly do that. It's not necessary, though.] ... ...

... ... Feel the reminder card consciously between your fingers and if you want, open your eyes briefly and look at the card ... ... open your eyes and read what it says ... ... I embrace life ... ... Now close your eyes again and let the read words resonate deeply within you ... ... deeply ... ...

You still feel the card between your fingers ... ... You know it can remind you every day to embrace your life ... ... Whenever you take the card in your hand and read it, you immediately feel freer and calmer inside ... ... freer and calmer ... ... Whenever you carry the card with you, you feel calmer and freer inside ... ... calmer and freer ... ... It happens naturally because your inner self knows that this card reminds you of what you have committed to today ... ... I embrace life ... ...

#4

Grief and Unresolved Conflicts

The following hypnosis session works with a combination of affirmation hypnosis and anchor technique. An affirmation is a short belief statement offered as a suggestion and can be used by the client as self-suggestion. An anchor is a trigger that evokes a specific feeling or thought. We work with the affirmation and simultaneously with an anchor in the form of a handy card with the printed phrase "I embrace life". This short phrase is an excerpt from the affirmation. We aim to help the client quickly adjust to letting go of grief and actively embracing life with the help of a "reminder card" when they notice that grief is holding them back in everyday life. We discuss this with the client before the session and prepare the reminder card. It can be a labeled business card or something similar. The card is prepared and given to the client. They can hold it loosely in their hand or place it on their body, for example on the solar plexus, during the hypnosis. The card should be carried by the client after the hypnosis, in their pants or jacket pocket. The main hypnosis part is deliberately kept very short to make the affirmation very clear and establish it as a fundamental statement, as a new belief. The advantage of hypnosis is that the affirmation is more easily accepted by the client than in a conscious state. However, this hypnosis should not serve as the first session but should be introduced when the client has already gone through a certain processing stage.

You are here today because someone has died with whom you had unresolved issues ... ... So much was left unsaid ... ... unresolved ... ... There were things you wanted to address but were unable to ... ... Sometimes you feel guilty and think you could have managed it all if you had just tackled it ... ... At the same time, you realize that you can still resolve everything that matters to you within yourself ... ... It's primarily about finding your inner peace ... ... embracing life ... ... Today, you can achieve something special ... ... Today, you can find peace and thereby embrace life again ... ... You have already dealt with yourself and your past, also with the fact that you have mourned for the person you miss ... ... also with the fact that you mourn for what is no longer possible ... ... This grief is an important feeling ... ... When you feel it, you can allow it and then let it go ... ...

... ... Perhaps you think that the conflict you had with him/her can no longer be easily addressed or resolved ... ... But it can be done ... ... Today, you can do something much more important than fighting out a conflict ... ... Today, you can choose to accept that the conflict existed instead of resolving it ... ... We often learn more from conflicts than from things that go smoothly ... ... So, today you fully commit to letting go ... ... to forgoing the resolution of the conflict ... ... to forgoing reparation or revenge ... ... to forgoing balance and reconciliation ... ... instead, to reconcile with yourself internally ... ... Truly remarkable how well you succeed in this today ... ... impressive how well you can adjust to letting go today and finding peace in that ... ...

Breathe deeply in and out ... ... deeply in ... ... and slowly and long out ... ... [in the client's breathing rhythm, please] ... ... and once more deeply in ... ... and out ... ... in ... ... and out ... ...

Now think of the person who has passed away ... ... Imagine this person is now with you and then speak to this person ... ... Repeat after me in your thoughts, if you want, you can also whisper it ... ...

I embrace life,

at the cost it has taken me

and the cost it has taken you.

Good can and will come from this.

None of this will be in vain.

You let the words resonate deeply within you and continue to look at the person ... ... Look into their face ... ... Then say again ... ...

I embrace life,

at the cost it has taken me

and the cost it has taken you.

Good can and will come from this.

None of this will be in vain.

You know the crucial phrase ... ... I embrace life ... ... It is like a message to yourself ... ... I embrace life ... ... You have this card with exactly this inscription, the card that holds your task ... ... I embrace life ... ...

... ... [Now ask the client to open their eyes and read the sentence while in trance. This reinforces the effect. Opening the eyes is a fractionation, but it can be done without specific announcement or counting. Everyone can open their eyes in trance. In a stable and deep trance, it is a bit cumbersome because the client is tired and sluggish. Just stay with suggestive encouragement until the eyes are opened and the card is read. If you prefer to initiate the fractionation by counting, you can certainly do that. It's not necessary, though.] ... ...

... ... Feel the reminder card consciously between your fingers and if you want, open your eyes briefly and look at the card ... ... open your eyes and read what it says ... ... I embrace life ... ... Now close your eyes again and let the read words resonate deeply within you ... ... deeply ... ...

#5

You are here today to say goodbye ... ... Death has separated you from a loved one ... ... [If possible, directly address who has died ... separated from your wife ... from your father, etc.] ... ... Sometimes we have time to prepare for death while the person is still alive because we know it is approaching ... ... with serious illnesses, we confront it ... ... In many cases, it happens so quickly and unexpectedly that we had no time to prepare ... ... could not say goodbye or even prepare for a farewell ... ... But finally, it is almost always the case that we did not manage to say goodbye beforehand because we held on ... ... because it only becomes final when death separates us ... ... Probably a farewell is never really easy ... ...

Today, however, you can do something that helps you both let go and hold on to loving memories ... ... Memories that can help you repeatedly to look back lovingly on the past to draw hope and courage from it ... ... At the same time, you must let go because the shared path in our world has ended ... ...

So today you think back to honor what you shared once more ... ... to let go of the unfinished, if there is anything unfinished ... ... and to say what has not been said ... ... or simply what you still want to say ... ...

Deep within you, you have photos of all the people you know ... ... like a huge album in your memory ... ... a gallery of your life so far ... ... All the situations and events ... ... all experiences ... ... even wishes and fantasies are stored deep within you ... ... and whenever you think of a specific event or a certain person, you can hold a matching photo in your hand ... ...

So now you find a photo of the loved one who has passed away ... [a photo of your husband ... a photo of your wife ...] ... ... The photo shows a very typical image, just as you most often saw this person ... ... You look at the photo ... ... As you do, memories come alive within you ... ... You recall what it was like when you first consciously met ... ... perhaps just a brief moment of attention that brought you together ... ... or simply fate that wanted it that way ... ... The images of memory come alive ... ... It is as if you were in that past time ... ... could experience again as a visitor what it was like back then ... ...

Then you find a photo from stormy and challenging times ... ... The photo shows that you experienced a lot together ... ... there were also arguments and conflicts ... ... perhaps openly fought ... ... or silently within yourself ... ... But then you managed, and better times came again ... ... You never lost each other, no, you always found each other again ... ... are connected to each other ... ...

You find a photo from the best time you spent together ... ... This photo comes to life naturally ... ... It is as if you can now immerse yourself in that time once more ... ... You are a visitor in that time and let the atmosphere of that time affect you again ... ... You feel it and experience the good feeling of shared experiences and events once more, the beautiful time ... ... But perhaps every time was beautiful in its own way ... ... Everything has its meaning and every challenge teaches us ... ... Look at everything in peace and enjoy the beautiful time once more ... ... the beautiful experiences ... ... if you want, choose a very special experience ... ... and look at it again in peace ... ... Let all the feelings and moods simply be there ... ... All of this belongs to you ... ...

... [Give about a minute of perceived time, then continue reading.] ...

Then a very special photo falls into your hand ... ... one that has a very special and personal meaning ... ... It appears naturally ... ... Accept it, whatever this photo shows ... ... You know why this particular image comes to mind ... ... You associate it with a deep inner feeling ... ... Let this feeling be fully present ... ... If you now pay attention to your feelings, you can sense the deep connection to the person who has left you ... ... There is surely something you want to say ... ... You can do this now deeply within yourself, just for you ... ... quietly ... ...say everything you still want to say now, until you hear my voice again ... ...

... ... [Now give about 2-3 minutes of perceived time and remain silent.] ... ...

You hear my voice again, because I am still here with you ... ... You have now used the time to speak or say deeply within yourself what you still wanted to say ... ... If you need a moment longer, then finish it ... ... continue speaking within yourself ... ... In a few moments, we will continue ... ...

... [Give the client another half minute, then continue reading.] ...

Now you have said everything important ... ... Now it is time to say goodbye ... ... to say farewell and slowly prepare to return to your wakeful everyday life ... ... You can now shake hands or give a final hug to the person who is with you ... [your husband ... your wife ... your father ...] ...

Now it is time to move on ... ... You know that you can always look deeply into yourself again in a state of calm and view the photos of your memories again ... ... So, you can say goodbye again and again ... ... just like today ... ... again and again, just like today ... ...

#6

Grief and Guilt after Surviving an Accident with Fatalities

You survived ... ... You were involved in this serious accident and could have died, just like the others did ... ... But you survived, and perhaps you have often thought that it would be fitting if you could be happy about it ... ... Yet you haven't been able to develop that feeling so far ... ... You survived, but it seems as if a part of you died ... ... as if you are sharing the fate of the others ... ...

But you know that's not possible ... ... Your task now is to keep living ... ... to make the best out of the challenges of your life ... ... to recognize what has been given to you despite all the pain ... ... life ... ... You had so many dreams and ideas before the accident ... ... intentions and plans ... ... goals in your life ... ... You can still achieve these goals because you are still here ... ... You want to find strength for that ... ... and soon regain new joy in life to enjoy your life again ... ... to be able to see your survival as a gift ... ... Seeing and accepting this gift is possible when you can also allow yourself to grieve ... ... Grieve for the people who died in this accident … … Grieve that such a terrible event happened at all … …

… … So today, you resolve to accomplish two things … … to mourn for the people who died in this accident … … and to accept your own life that is open to you and waiting for you … …

… … Deep within you, there is a place we call the Place of Clarity … … It is a place where you can see everything clearly … … understand everything well … … and best encounter yourself … … Everything becomes clear at this inner place … … Everything becomes understandable at this inner place … … Everything becomes good at this inner place … … Today, you can find this place within yourself … … Breathe deeply into your center … … Imagine how the oxygen you breathe in flows deeply into you and gathers in the center of your body, where the solar plexus is … … Breathe calmly and evenly and follow the flow of your breath … … Follow your breath into your solar plexus … … over and over again … … As you do, you sink deeper and deeper into your feelings … … Let it become quieter and darker and immerse yourself in your feelings … … It becomes darker and darker and quieter and quieter … … darker and darker and quieter and quieter ... ... darker and darker and quieter and quieter ... ... And deep within you, you find this light that becomes brighter and brighter ... ... with each breath, the light deep inside you becomes brighter and clearer ... ... brighter and clearer ... ... brighter and clearer ... ... with each breath brighter and clearer until only white, pure light surrounds you ... ... You are completely surrounded by pure white light ... ... enveloped in white, pure light ... ... You have arrived at the Place of Clarity ... ...

At this place, there is only white, pure light ... ... You stand at this place and see only light all around you ... ... Let this vision become very clear ... ... white light around you ... ... only light everywhere ... ... Immerse yourself fully in the vision of pure white light and complete inner freedom ... ...

The ground beneath your feet seems glassy ... ... you can see through it ... ... infinitely deep ... ... But even there, you only see pleasant, white light ... ... You look up and see only light above you as well ... ... It is everywhere ... ... bright and clear and very pleasant ... ... It envelops you and gives you clarity and openness ... ... You see a glass wall in front of you ... ... You can see through it and see only light behind the wall as well ... ... It is beautiful at the Place of Clarity ...

... so pure ... ... so free ... ... so bright and clear ... ... so distinct ... ... You look once more at the glass wall in front of you ... ... On the other side of the wall are the people who did not survive the accident ... ... They look peaceful and unscathed ... ... They radiate an incredible calm ... ...

You stand very close to the wall ... ... You can see them ... ... They speak to you ... ... You can hear their voices ... ... The deceased thank you because you thought about them so much with your inner struggle ... ... always wondering why they had to die and why you survived ... ... They thank you for this empathy and tell you at the same time that you have thought of them and mourned enough ... ... They tell you that you are innocent and that there is a reason you are still alive ... ... It is now up to you to find or rediscover this reason ... ... You survived ... ... You survived ... ...

... ... Then you breathe deeply in and slowly and long out, letting go of your guilt ... ... and again ... ... breathe in ... [in the client's breathing rhythm, please] ... and breathe out ... [Extend the word "out," slightly longer than the client's actual exhalation, to slow their breathing and lengthen the exhalation.] ... breathe in ... ... breathe out ... ... and let go ... ... breathe in ... ... breathe out ... ... and let go ... ...

It gets darker deep inside you; you slowly fade out the images within you ... ... Each additional breath helps you let go of your old guilt feelings even more and better accept your own life ... ... You accept your life ... ... And every day, when you give yourself peace and close your eyes to breathe consciously and slowly, your inner self remembers to let go of guilt and accept life ... ... every day just like today ... ... just like today ... ...

#7

The following application can be done without a trance induction and is therefore all the more emphatic. An arm catalepsy (immobility of the outstretched arm) is set up, symbolizing the holding on to grief and the associated inner immobility, the standstill. The reversal of the catalepsy stands as a symbol for freeing oneself from holding on and thus overcoming grief and unfulfillable longing for the past. Symbolically, inner mobility returns with the external resolution of the catalepsy. Of course, the whole thing can also be done after an extensive trance induction, but I recommend refraining from that because the functioning catalepsy without (prepared) hypnosis leaves a more lasting impression. Experienced hypnotists know: catalepsy works without hypnosis, but when it works, it is hypnosis!

You probably can't just read the following text as you would with all the others. I still want to encourage you to try this variant once. It's not about the wording but the procedure. You don't have to memorize every word.

I want to show you that your feeling of not being able to continue living or feeling joy alone is largely an ingrained belief. A belief you can let go of to overcome your grief. Your grief had a purpose, but that purpose is now fulfilled. You have dealt with yourself and death, understood a lot, and perhaps some things remain unresolved. Maybe you wanted to say or clarify something important before death separated you. Perhaps you think you should have done some things differently in hindsight. But everything had its meaning and its time. Something always remains unresolved when a person dies. That is why we often hold on to the memory and our guilt feelings in grief so strongly that we believe we can no longer live joyfully. We consider it impossible. This is often because we have ordered ourselves not to be happy or cheerful anymore. If we allow ourselves to keep living, we can also overcome great losses.

But you believe that it is no longer possible to live joyfully. I claim that this feeling is there because you can't imagine that it can go away or change. You probably also can't imagine that you wouldn't be able to move your arm anymore just because you suddenly imagine that it can't be moved. You probably don't believe that. Alright. I want to show you something that can demonstrate your own thinking. The thinking deep inside you. The unconscious thinking. But you can influence that too. I will help you with that.

Catalepsy Phase

Now stretch out your right arm straight ... [Make sure the arm is stretched out and held horizontally forward; use the left for left-handed people] ... Now find a point on your hand and fix your gaze on it, for example, a knuckle. Keep your focus on this point. Now imagine that this arm is getting longer and longer. It stretches longer and longer. Look at your knuckle. The arm becomes two meters long, three meters long. Longer and longer. Imagine it. Your arm becomes five meters long, ten meters long. Longer and longer. It becomes even a hundred meters long. And it becomes firmer and more stable. The longer it gets, the firmer your arm becomes. Your arm becomes two hundred meters long. A kilometer. Look at the knuckle. Your arm stretches, becoming longer, ten kilometers long. It drills through the city. And now imagine that your arm becomes firmer the longer it gets and let it become even longer. Imagine that every attempt to move your arm makes it a kilometer longer. And firmer. As soon as you try to push your upper arm down, your arm becomes a kilometer longer and firmer. You now try to push your upper arm down, and your arm stretches ... Once again. Try to push your upper arm down, and your arm stretches ... Try it again, and your arm becomes longer and firmer ... ... Try it again. Your arm stays firm ... ...

This simple exercise can also be used as a suggestibility test. It works very well and is really doable in a short time without prior trance induction. It doesn't take more than one or two minutes until the arm remains straight and firm upon the request to push it down. Simple but effective suggestion!

It doesn't work anymore. You can't do both at the same time. Moving and becoming firmer doesn't work. Your belief that your arm is becoming longer and firmer keeps it horizontal. If I now tell you that this isn't true, that you just combined two incompatible things, you can imagine that your arm will immediately become short and movable upon the next attempt to move it. Your arm is movable. You just need to know it. Your arm is completely movable. Move your arm.

Distribution, publication, and copying in any form are prohibited and subject to damages.

Copying, publishing, and sharing with third parties are only permitted with the written consent of the author. Please observe the notes on copyright and usage.

Now discuss this exercise with your client. Explain to them that their grief and guilt feelings are similar. They believe they are unchangeable, immovable like the cataleptic arm, and that they can't influence them. Repeat the exercise and let the client speak. They should hold the outstretched arm and say repeatedly: "My arm is getting longer and firmer." Check the catalepsy for them by applying light pressure to the arm. Let them say several times: "When I try to move my arm, it gets firmer." They should then try. Initially, this will likely lead to catalepsy, which they should then resolve themselves by saying: "I can and will now move my arm because it is movable!" Practice a bit with the client until they manage to establish and resolve catalepsy themselves.

Dear readers, try this exercise at least once. It is fun and usually brings an "aha effect." It shows that belief can work very quickly and clearly in one direction and then also in the other direction. Try the exercise on yourself. You will be surprised how well it works in self-suggestion and how quickly you can cancel the effect. Of course, you can prevent the effect from the beginning. Please try it out ...

#8

You have experienced the painful end of a shared path that was ended by death ... ... A loved one has died ... [It is better to name the person ... Your friend has died ... Your mother has died ...] ...and your thoughts are still attached to him/her. You try to process everything that has happened and prepare yourself internally to both process and let go ... ... Because the shared path in this life has now ended ... ... You know it is not easy to just move on and leave the grief behind ... ... But it is possible ... ... You can do it ... ... here and today ... ...

You delve deeper and deeper into your own feelings ... ... With each breath, you go deeper into relaxation ... ... You breathe into your inner center, into your solar plexus, and find calm ... ... Calm is something you can really use right now ... ...

You think back to the good times you had ... ... You remember how good everything once felt ... ... You know that you were able to enjoy many things in your shared life, on your shared path ... ... Images of your memories pass before your inner eye and bring back the good feelings ... ... Your body responds to these pleasant memories ... ... perhaps you notice that your body changes with your thoughts ... ... When you think of something good, your body takes on a pleasant posture ... ... just like now ... ... pleasantly calm and with a constructive tension ... ... The deeper you now dive into the beautiful memories, the better your body can remember and take on this positive posture ... ... You can also recall other beautiful memories, even ones unrelated to this relationship ... ... beautiful images of your good memories, so you can now inform your body how good you once felt ... ... Your body adopts this good posture now ... ... Your body adopts this posture now and shows you with its pleasant position that you can feel even better ... ... right now ... ... Just like that, it is right ... ... It works, and therefore you can make the pleasant feeling even better now ... ... just like that ... ... exactly like that ... ... Your body stores the best posture and the most constructive tension it can take on to help you come into a strong and constructive position repeatedly ... ... Then you think of the separation by death, maybe of difficult moments or phases you had on your shared path ... ... You recall these images internally and immediately remember the painful and sorrowful feelings ... ... Your body takes on these positions too ... ... Maybe you have already noticed that your breathing has changed ... ... the tension of your muscles ... ... the position of your body ... ... Your body follows your thoughts ... ... Even if you now have unpleasant feelings, let them become clear, make them conscious, because they are part of you ... ... Every feeling within you has its justification ... ... Let your feelings be there because you can benefit most from them this way ... ... This way, you can overcome grief and pain the fastest ... ... Now immerse yourself completely in your feelings ... ...

... [Give about a minute of perceived time, then continue reading.] ...

Now imagine white light ... ... Imagine you are surrounded only by light, and everything becomes bright around you ... ... Your body now lets go of all tension ... ... You become calmer and calmer ... ... with each breath calmer ... ... You let go and become calm ... ... You let go and become calm ... ... Your muscles relax, your breathing becomes calm ... ... Your body comes to rest, and so do your thoughts ... ... Your thoughts become even calmer ... ... In your inner center, the feeling of freedom arises ... ... You want to go new ways ... ... The past is past ... ... Now you start anew ... ... right now ... ... Your body now takes on the best position to move forward with strength and joy ... ... Your body makes all its energy available to you and corrects your posture ... ... You take on the outer posture that is suitable to move forward with strength and leave the past behind ... ... Your head takes the best position ... ... Your shoulders align ... ... Your arms take a strong posture ... ... Your hands get ready to grasp ... ... Your upper body takes the position that helps you to move forward constructively, to conquer the world ... ... Your belly and back take on a posture that allows your upper body to be carried upright and proud ... ... Your breathing becomes strong and wide ... ... Your legs receive the signal to be strong, to carry your body securely, upright and stable ... ... Your feet get ready to carry the weight of your body securely and keep it stable ... ... You observe yourself as in a mirror and see that your body has taken an upright and proud position ... ... Let this image become clear ... ... Your body increasingly adopts this posture ... ... This posture becomes deeply ingrained in you because it helps you today and every day ... ... today and every day ... ...

Today you let go of your grief … … You preserve the memory, but you let go of the grief … …

Your body increasingly adjusts to promote your good feelings … … Your deep inner self memorizes the best posture for this very precisely and helps you every day to come into a strong and constructive posture … … This makes your feelings of strength, your curiosity about life, and your forward-looking attitude ever stronger … …

#9

You often think about a deceased person because you miss them so much ... [In a group, use general phrases like here in the text; in individual sessions, it is better to personalize the text, e.g., ... about your deceased mother, whom you miss ...] ... perhaps about many things that remained unsaid, many things you had planned with the person ... [your mother ... your friend ...] ... but can no longer experience ... ... The longing remains, but you know it can no longer be fulfilled because it is no longer possible ... ... This has often made you sad ... ... So the desire has arisen to overcome your grief and let go ... ... to come to terms with the fact that your paths have separated ... ... to accept it and make your peace with it ... ... perhaps even more ... ... because it is also possible to keep the beautiful memories and still live your life in peace ... ...

You prepare for an inner journey ... ... a journey to a distant land that is also very close ... ... the land of your dreams ... ... Feel the rhythm of your breathing and follow it

… … With the wind of your breath, you leave your thoughts and go to the land of dreams … …

You stand before the entrance of an old castle … … It stands at the edge of the forest and looks like it is many hundreds of years old … … At the same time, it seems familiar to you … … You feel like you have been here before … … So you go very close … … climb the steps and open the heavy dark wooden door, which opens very easily … … and full of trust, almost as if by itself, you go inside … … You close the door behind you … …

… … Inside, you notice that mirrors hang on the walls everywhere … … The mirrors sparkle and shine beautifully … … they reflect the light … … You follow the wide hallway through the castle and open the door at the end of the corridor … … You go through it and come into a large room … … It is huge, and you walk all the way through it … … At the end, you find a door that gives you access to the next large room … … So you go from room to room until you find the right room … … the room of your memories … …

All your life memories are here in this room … … Here nothing can be lost … … Here, too, mirrors hang on the walls everywhere ... ... When you look into a mirror, you see images of your own memory ... ... Images you often remember ... ... also images you had almost forgotten ... ... They come naturally ... ... show themselves before your inner eye and mirror what occupies you deep inside ... ... You look into the mirror of shared places ... ... You see there in the mirror images of special places ... ... places you both liked to be together ... ... perhaps vacation spots ... ... perhaps favorite places very close to you ... ... and also places from everyday life ... ... a favorite armchair ... ... or a window you looked out of together ... ... Whatever your shared places may be, wherever your shared places were ... ... You see them here and feel the connection that existed between you and still exists ... ...

You preserve the memory, and at the same time, you move on ... ... You look into a mirror that shows you shared interests ... ... You see in the mirror what topics and activities you both ... [or: your friend and you, etc.] ... liked ... ... can once again observe how it was some time ago ... ... Perhaps you also find interests from earlier times that are long ago, but they also belong to you and your history ... ...

You preserve the memory, and at the same time, you move on ... ...

Finally, you look into the mirror of plans ... ... You see images of the plans and projects you could no longer carry out together ... ... death has separated you, so some ideas had to remain unfulfilled ... ... Perhaps there were even old plans you had wanted to realize for a long time or repeatedly ... ... But now that is no longer possible ... ... You see them here and feel the connection that existed between you and still exists ... ... You preserve the memory, and at the same time, you move on ... ... Then you go to the center of the room and let all your feelings affect you ... ... You consciously perceive your feelings and let them be ... ... You also feel the sensations of your body ... ... It shows you how your deep emotions feel because your inner self sends them out as bodily sensations ... ... You immerse yourself completely in the world of your feelings ... ... Then you open all the windows in this room ... ... You also go into the adjacent rooms and throw all the windows open ... ... Wind flows through the rooms ... ... You feel a warm wind blowing through the rooms ... ... It helps you to feel lighter inside at this moment ... ... The wind carries away all your burdens and all your troubling thoughts and blows over the land of dreams ... ... It frees and cleanses you inside ... ... You feel free ... ...

You go back to the long castle hallway and find the exit ... ... You go outside and close the door behind you ... ...

You say goodbye to all the images and impressions ... ... You can visit this time again in your memory at any time ... ... But now you continue alone on this path in this life ... ... until you meet again one day. You go outside, at your speed, at your pace ... ... and close the door ... ... You must move on ... ... You think about how the land of dreams is deep inside you. It has always been there. I'm just telling you about it ... ...

#10

Death of a Pet

You prepare for an inner journey ... ... a journey to a distant land that is also very close ... ... the land of your dreams ... ... In this land, anything is possible that can also happen in your imagination ... . And here, there is space just for you ... ... just for you ... ...

You go to the land of dreams ... ... You are here to finally give space to your grief ... ... finally to be in your feelings without judgment and without evaluation ... ... You grieve for an animal that was like a friend to you, more than that: a love ... ... You know that people can feel as much for animals as for other people ... ... You had perhaps more connected with your animal ... [your dog ... your cat ... your horse ...] ... than with many people who think they are close to you ... ... Your feeling is your feeling, and you feel it now just as it is ... ... if you feel it, it can change again ... ... But today, your feeling gets all the space in the land of dreams ... ... and this land is infinitely large ... ... infinitely large ... ...

You are sitting in the middle of a beautiful green meadow ... ... You look up into the sky, and the weather is just the way you like it best ... ... Maybe you like the sun, then it should be a beautiful sunny day ... ... pleasantly warm ... ... or you love the wind ... ... then you can feel it on your skin ... ... However you like it best, that is how it should be in the land of your dreams ... ... You lie down ... ... You make yourself comfortable and look at the sky, which becomes a huge screen ... ...

The clouds slowly move aside like a curtain opening ... ... And in big letters, it says in the sky: YOU HAVE THE RIGHT TO GRIEVE ... ... Exactly this right you take for yourself here and today ... ... You let your feelings flow through the land of dreams ... ... The wind carries it everywhere ... ... your grief ... ... your longing ... ... your despair ... ... whatever feelings you have, they flow like warm wind through the land of dreams ... ... your land ... ... Your feelings are a part of you ... ... The further your feelings flow through the land of dreams, the lighter you feel ... ... with each breath lighter ... ... and lighter ... ...

You look at the sky, and new writings keep appearing that you can read ... ... Next, it says: LOVE IS A FEELING ... ... It reminds you that this is exactly what you feel for your animal ... [your dog ... your cat ... your horse ...] ... Love ... ... Not everyone has always understood this ... ... You know the feeling of love for a person, but also the feeling of love for your animal ... [your dog ... your cat ... your horse ...] ... So you let this feeling become very intense again ... ... the beautiful feeling of affection and connection ... ... Then you think of the love of your animal for you ... [your dog ... your cat ... your horse ...] ... It was always unconditional ... ... always unbroken ... ... An animal does not differentiate between rich and poor ... ... between right and wrong in your actions ... ... It never judges your mood or impatience ... ... It shares your condition with you ... ... and sometimes reflects you ... ... Then you have seen yourself in the behavior and reactions of your animal ... ...

... [Give about half a minute of perceived time, then continue reading.] ...

You look at the sky and see the words: YOUR TEARS ARE HERE ... ... As you ponder the meaning of these words, it begins to rain ... ... Salty raindrops fall on your face ... ... They taste like your own tears ... ... the tears you have already cried ... ... the tears you may have suppressed ... ...

the tears you perhaps did not want to show because you could not allow them ... ... Maybe you know the thought, the inner question, whether it is right to grieve so much for an animal as you do ... ... Wherever this hesitation may come from ... ... It does not come from your heart ... ... From your heart comes the feeling of love ... ... the pain of loss ... ... the desire to hold your animal in your arms again ... ... to be with it once more ... ... to tell it how much you love it ... ...

... [Give about half a minute of perceived time, then continue reading.] ...

Then you see the words in the sky: I KNOW WHAT YOU FEEL ... ... A greeting from your deceased animal ... ... now living in the land beyond the rainbow and knowing exactly what you feel ... ... It has long forgiven you if you were less able to care for it at times because you had other difficulties and burdens ... ... It has long forgiven you if you were ever rough or impatient or did anything else you now see as a mistake ... ... In fact, it did not even need to forgive you because it was never angry with you ... ... never blamed you ... ... Your animal always lived in the moment and could always let go of the past ... ...

Now you must let go ... ... but only the shared path on earth ... ... And eventually your pain ... ... Then you will live in the moment, just like your beloved animal ... ... You close your eyes and rest on the meadow ... ... in the land of dreams ... ... You allow yourself to grieve ... ... You allow yourself to feel pain ... ... You allow yourself to cry ... ... Then you think about how the land of dreams is deep inside you ... ... It has always been there ... ... I am just telling you about it ...

Overview of All Titles in the Series "Ten Hypnoses"

Volume 1: Smoking Cessation
Volume 2: Anxiety and Restlessness
Volume 3: Burnout
Volume 4: Reducing Overweight
Volume 5: Coping with the Past
Volume 6: Suicidal Thoughts and Attempts
Volume 7: Psycho-Oncology
Volume 8: Obsessions and Tics
Volume 9: Self-Confidence and Decision-Making
Volume 10: Grief Work
Volume 11: Psychosomatics
Volume 12: Chronic Pain
Volume 13: Depressive Thoughts
Volume 14: Panic Attacks
Volume 15: Domestic Violence, Victim Support
Volume 16: Post-Traumatic Stress
Volume 17: Exam Anxiety and Stage Fright
Volume 18: Anti-Violence Training, Offender Support
Volume 19: Addiction Tendencies
Volume 20: Social Phobia and Fear of Contact
Volume 21: Nail Biting
Volume 22: Self-Awareness and Self-Love
Volume 23: Teeth Grinding and Night Clenching
Volume 24: Feelings of Guilt
Volume 25: Fear in Crowds
Volume 26: Fear of Flying, Aviophobia
Volume 27: Fear in Enclosed Spaces, Claustrophobia
Volume 28: Tinnitus, Ear Noises
Volume 29: Fear of Heights
Volume 30: Neurodermatitis

Copying, publishing, and sharing with third parties are only permitted with the written consent of the author. Please observe the notes on copyright and usage.

Volume 31: Finding Inner Balance
Volume 32: Overcoming Loneliness
Volume 33: Fear of Illness, Hypochondria
Volume 34: Anticipatory Anxiety, Fear of Fear
Volume 35: Jealousy in Relationships
Volume 36: Driving Anxiety
Volume 37: New Start after Separation
Volume 38: Fear of Injections
Volume 39: Heart Anxiety Neurosis
Volume 40: Overcoming Resentment and Anger
Volume 41: Resolving Blockages and Positive Thinking
Volume 42: Stress Reduction, Stress Management
Volume 43: Body Relaxation
Volume 44: Deep Relaxation
Volume 45: Fear of the Dark
Volume 46: Falling Asleep and Staying Asleep
Volume 47: Compulsive Buying
Volume 48: Restless Legs Syndrome
Volume 49: Bulimia
Volume 50: Anorexia
Volume 51: Overcoming Nightmares
Volume 52: Imagined Deformity
Volume 53: Overcoming Distrust, Finding Trust
Volume 54: Processing Failures
Volume 55: Humiliation, Emotional Hurt
Volume 56: Distressing Compassion, Vicarious Suffering
Volume 57: Self-Forgiveness
Volume 58: Self-Awareness, Self-Confidence
Volume 59: Saying No
Volume 60: Assertiveness
Volume 61: Setting Boundaries and Self-Assertion
Volume 62: Decision-Making Ability

Volume 63: Success Orientation
Volume 64: Ruminating, Circular Thinking
Volume 65: Accepting Pregnancy
Volume 66: Birth Preparation
Volume 67: Spiritual Opening
Volume 68: Joy of Life and Inner Lightness
Volume 69: Patience and Inner Peace
Volume 70: Fibromyalgia and Rheumatism
Volume 71: Irritable Bowel Syndrome, Crohn's Disease
Volume 72: Fear of Nausea, Emetophobia
Volume 73: Stuttering and Cluttering, Speech Flow Disorders
Volume 74: Concentration and Knowledge Anchoring
Volume 75: Vitality and Spontaneity
Volume 76: Searching for Meaning and Finding Goals
Volume 77: Life Crises, Life Events
Volume 78: Workaholism, Goal Obsession
Volume 79: Helper Syndrome, Helpless Helpers
Volume 80: Medication Abuse
Volume 81: Gambling Addiction
Volume 82: Internet Addiction, Smartphone Addiction
Volume 83: Hoarding Disorder, Compulsive Collecting
Volume 84: Conspiracy Thoughts, Overvalued Ideas
Volume 85: Fear of Operations and Treatments
Volume 86: Fear of Aging
Volume 87: Travel Anxiety
Volume 88: Anxiety When Urinating, Paruresis
Volume 89: Fear of Intimacy and Togetherness
Volume 90: Fear of Blushing
Volume 91: Coming Out in Homosexuality
Volume 92: Charisma Training
Volume 93: Migraines and Chronic Headaches
Volume 94: Overcoming Allergies, Bronchial Asthma

Volume 95: Normalizing Blood Pressure
Volume 96: Compulsive Perfectionism
Volume 97: Sports Hypnosis, Motivation
Volume 98: Sports Hypnosis, Performance Enhancement
Volume 99: Determination and Focus
Volume 100: Encountering the Inner Child
Volume 101: Cravings, Binge Eating
Volume 102: Stimulating Metabolism
Volume 103: Bipolar Mood Swings
Volume 104: Borderline, Identity Crises
Volume 105: Hypomania, Euphoria, Mania
Volume 106: Restlessness, Agitation
Volume 107: Nervous Breakdown
Volume 108: Adjustment Disorders
Volume 109: Self-Alienation, Depersonalization
Volume 110: Ending Self-Pity
Volume 111: Primary Gain of Illness
Volume 112: Secondary Gain of Illness
Volume 113: Bullying, Victim Support
Volume 114: Letting Go of Envy and Jealousy
Volume 115: Fear of Spiders, Arachnophobia
Volume 116: Fear of Dogs or Cats
Volume 117: Fear of Strangers, Xenophobia
Volume 118: Excessive Worries, Generalized Anxiety
Volume 119: Strengthening Sense of Responsibility
Volume 120: Unrequited Love, Heartache
Volume 121: Work-Life Balance
Volume 122: Letting Go of Unattainable Goals
Volume 123: Allowing and Accepting Help
Volume 124: Letting Go of Adult Children
Volume 125: Tourette Syndrome
Volume 126: Life Changes and New Starts

Volume 127: Accepting Life in a Wheelchair
Volume 128: Understanding and Overcoming Homesickness
Volume 129: Understanding and Overcoming Wanderlust
Volume 130: Dizziness, Meniere's Disease
Volume 131: Overcoming Aggression
Volume 132: Cutting and Self-Harm
Volume 133: Hair Pulling, Trichotillomania
Volume 134: Postpartum Depression
Volume 135: For Relatives of Dementia Patients
Volume 136: Self-Harm, Artificial Disorders
Volume 137: Activating Self-Healing Powers
Volume 138: Preventing Depression Relapse
Volume 139: Reactive Psychoses, Follow-Up
Volume 140: Obsessive Thoughts and Impulses
Volume 141: Compulsive Checking
Volume 142: Compulsive Counting, Symmetry Obsession
Volume 143: Compulsive Washing, Cleanliness Obsession
Volume 144: Compulsive Questioning
Volume 145: Dissociative Paralysis
Volume 146: Phantom Pain
Volume 147: Overcoming Complaining
Volume 148: Hay Fever, Pollen Allergy
Volume 149: Sexual Abuse, Victim Support
Volume 150: Standing Strong Against Sexism, #metoo
Volume 151: Binge Eating
Volume 152: Overcoming Thoughts of Revenge
Volume 153: Detachment from the Aggressor, Stockholm Syndrome
Volume 154: Courage to Separate
Volume 155: Chronic Fatigue, Exhaustion
Volume 156: Fear of the Future, Existential Anxiety
Volume 157: Excessive Worry About Children
Volume 158: Fear of Failure

Volume 159: Ending Distrust and Control
Volume 160: Dejection, Dysphoria
Volume 161: Boreout, Chronic Boredom
Volume 162: Bipolar Disorders, Relapse Prevention
Volume 163: Mania, Relapse Prevention
Volume 164: Nihilism, Feelings of Worthlessness
Volume 165: Thumb Sucking
Volume 166: Being Brave
Volume 167: Being Proud
Volume 168: Overcoming Shyness
Volume 169: Being Able to Delegate Responsibility
Volume 170: Being Able to Show Emotions
Volume 171: Letting Go of Guilt, Victim Support
Volume 172: Processing Guilt, Offender Support
Volume 173: Mood Swings, Cyclothymia
Volume 174: Lack of Drive, Vital Sadness
Volume 175: Hearing Voices with Reality Reference
Volume 176: Confident Communication
Volume 177: Standing Up for Oneself
Volume 178: Taking New Paths
Volume 179: Confident Job Application
Volume 180: No Longer Being Taken Advantage Of
Volume 181: End of Submissiveness
Volume 182: Depressive Numbness
Volume 183: Mood Drops, Affective Incontinence
Volume 184: Mood Instability
Volume 185: Somatoform Disorders
Volume 186: Stomach Ulcer, Psychosomatic
Volume 187: Accepting Amputation
Volume 188: Overcoming and Letting Go of Hatred
Volume 189: Ending Accusations
Volume 190: Allowing Tears, Being Able to Cry

Volume 191: Finding and Sorting Repressed Feelings
Volume 192: Somatoform Pain
Volume 193: Living Autonomously
Volume 194: Anhedonia, Joylessness
Volume 195: Persistent Sadness
Volume 196: Obesity, Food Addiction
Volume 197: Parents of Abused Children
Volume 198: Letting Go and Letting Be
Volume 199: Childhood Sexual Abuse
Volume 200: Fear of Loss

www.ingramcontent.com/pod-product-compliance
Lightning Source LLC
Chambersburg PA
CBHW030501220526
45464CB00006B/2600